Healthy Weight Loss After 60:

A Guide to Vitality and Longevity

By

Vanessa S. Castaneda

Table of Contents

Introduction

Welcome to "Healthy Weight Loss After 60: A Guide to Vitality and Longevity," your all-inclusive guide to achieving and keeping a healthy weight while appreciating the experience and vigor of your advanced age. We set out on a life-changing adventure to discover the secrets of healthy weight loss designed specifically for individuals over the age of 60 in this inspiring guide.

In today's age-obsessed world, the desire for a healthy weight frequently takes center stage. Achieving and maintaining a healthy weight after the age of 60 is not just about slipping into a smaller dress size; it's about valuing your health, vitality, and general well-being. That's why this book is more than simply a diet plan; it's a holistic approach to enjoying your best life as you age.

Throughout these pages, you will discover:

Understanding Your Body: Learn about the physiological changes that occur with aging and how they impact metabolism, body composition, and weight control. Learn about the specific problems and potential of weight loss after 60.

Mindful Eating: Learn how to create a healthy connection with food and develop mindful eating habits to help you lose weight. Discover how to navigate cravings, emotional eating, and social situations with grace and awareness.

Physical Activity: Enjoy the freedom of movement and learn about the numerous benefits of regular exercise for weight loss, strength, flexibility, and overall health. Explore a wide range of fitness options tailored to your level of fitness, interests, and skills.

Nutrition and Meal Planning: Explore tasty, nutrient-dense recipes and meal plans that will nourish your body, aid in healthy weight loss, and delight your taste buds. Learn how to make healthier food choices, plan balanced meals, and develop a long-term eating plan that works for you.

Lifestyle Factors: Investigate how sleep, stress management, hydration, and other lifestyle factors contribute to healthy weight loss and general wellness. Discover effective methods for improving your sleep quality, reducing stress, and prioritizing self-care.

As you embark on this journey of healthy weight loss after 60, remember that every positive decision you make to prioritize your health is a powerful investment in your vitality and life. By following the concepts outlined in this guide, you will be able to live a lively, meaningful life at any age.

Chapter 1: Understanding Weight Loss After 60

Introduction to How Metabolism Changes with Aging

Our bodily systems change dramatically as we get older, and one of the most significant shifts is in our metabolism. Metabolism is the process by which our bodies turn the foods we ingest into energy. This energy is required for everything from daily activities to maintaining basic bodily functions at rest, and it is referred to as our basal metabolic rate (BMR).

Several variables contribute to a decrease in metabolic rate with age:

1. **Reduced Muscle Mass**: Muscle tissue is more metabolically active than fat tissue. Sarcopenia is the slow loss of muscular mass that occurs with age, This loss occurs during our early 30s or 40s and accelerates with time, especially if we are not actively involved in resistance or

strength training to offset it. With lower muscle mass, our bodies need fewer calories to maintain weight, which can lead to weight gain if caloric intake is not adjusted.

2. **Hormonal Changes**: As we age, our hormones alter, which might affect our metabolism. Changes in the level of thyroid hormone, for instance, can decrease metabolic rate and make weight loss more difficult. Menopause causes a decrease in estrogen, which can contribute to weight gain, particularly around the abdomen. In men, levels of testosterone fall, which can lead to decreased muscle mass and a slower metabolism.

3. **Reduced Physical Activity**: As people age, they often become less physically active due to lifestyle changes, health challenges, or fears about injury. Reduced exercise decreases the metabolic rate even further because fewer calories are required for everyday functions.

4. **Changes in Energy Utilization**: As people get older, their bodies' energy usage may change. They may, for example, burn fewer calories when physically active than when at rest. Furthermore, as people age, their digestive systems become less efficient, affecting how nutrients are digested and used as energy.

The Significance of Weight Loss for Health After Age 60.

It is impossible to stress the importance of weight loss for health after 60. Weight management becomes an increasingly important aspect of general health maintenance and disease prevention as people age. Weight loss and maintaining a healthy weight are especially important after the age of 60 for the following reasons:

1. **Lower Risk of Chronic Diseases**: Being overweight can increase the risk of various chronic illnesses, including type 2

diabetes, heart disease, hypertension (high blood pressure), and some malignancies. Losing weight can help control or even prevent certain diseases, thereby improving longevity and quality of life.

2. **Increased Mobility and Independence**: Excess weight can place extra strain on joints, resulting in pain and disorders like osteoarthritis. Weight loss can reduce stress by improving mobility, thus increasing independence and the ability to complete everyday activities without assistance.

3. **Improved Arthritis and Joint Pain Management**: For people who already have arthritis, losing weight can help to lower the severity of their symptoms. For instance, losing one pound of weight can result in a fourfold decrease in the load placed on the knees, greatly reducing pain and improving joint function.

4. **Improved Respiratory Function**: Being overweight or obese can decrease respiratory function, making breathing

more difficult, even during modest exercises. Weight loss can increase lung function and oxygen efficiency, facilitating physical exercise and daily duties.

5. **Improved Metabolic Health**: Losing weight after 60 can boost insulin sensitivity, reduce inflammation, and lower the risk of metabolic syndrome. These modifications can significantly improve energy levels and overall health, making it simpler to lead an active and meaningful life.

6. **Increased Mental Health**: Weight loss and increased physical health can also have a favorable impact on mental health. Physical activity, a vital component of weight loss, causes the production of endorphins, which help to overcome stress, melancholy, and anxiety. Furthermore, meeting weight-loss objectives can increase self-esteem and confidence.

7. **Improved Sleep**: Overweight and obesity have been connected to sleep issues such as sleep apnea. Losing weight can improve sleep quality and length, boosting daily energy and cognitive performance.

8. **Longevity**: Studies have shown that maintaining a healthy weight can lead to a longer life expectancy. Weight loss can help extend one's life by reducing the risk of chronic diseases and increasing general physical and mental health.

Myths Concerning Weight Loss in Older Adults

Addressing common misconceptions about weight reduction among older people is crucial to guiding them through their health journey with accurate information and appropriate expectations. Here are some common myths, along with the reality behind them:

1. **Myth 1: Weight Loss is Impossible After a Specific Age**

Truth: Metabolism indeed slows with age, making weight loss more difficult, but it is not impossible. With the right diet, exercise, and lifestyle changes, older adults can successfully reduce weight. It may require more effort and patience than when they were younger, but it is certainly possible.

2. Myth 2: Older Adults Shouldn't Exercise Excessively

Truth: Physical activity is necessary for people of all ages, including those over 60. The key is determining the appropriate type and amount of exercise for an individual's health, mobility, and fitness level. Strength training, cardio, and flexibility activities can all be adapted for older adults and play an important part in weight management and overall health.

3. Myth 3: Reducing Calories Is the Key

Truth: While maintaining a calorie deficit is necessary for weight loss, the quality of the calories ingested is equally important.

Nutrient-dense foods, which contain vitamins, minerals, fiber, and protein, can benefit health in ways that empty calories from sugar and processed carbohydrates cannot. Proper nutrition also aids in hunger management and energy maintenance during exercise.

4. Myth 4: Losing Weight at My Age Won't Make Much Difference

Truth: Losing weight can have major health benefits at any age, including lowering the risk of chronic diseases, improving mobility, better managing pre-existing health conditions, and improving quality of life. Even small weight losses, such as 5% to 10% of body weight, can have a significant health impact.

5. Myth 5: I Need to Lose a Lot of Weight to See the Health Benefits

Truth: Small, lasting adjustments can result in significant health benefits. Moderate weight loss can improve blood pressure, cholesterol, and blood sugar levels, lowering the risk of chronic diseases associated with obesity.

6. Myth 6: Dieting Is the Most Effective Way to Weight

Truth: While diet plays an essential role in weight control, a multifaceted approach that includes regular physical activity, proper sleep, stress management, and social connections is more beneficial for long-term weight loss and health. "Dieting" in the classic sense can be unsustainable, resulting in a yo-yo diet cycle. Instead, concentrating on healthy eating habits throughout your life is key.

Chapter 2: The Nutritional Needs of Seniors

Important Nutrients and Their Sources for Elders

As individuals age, their dietary demands may shift, necessitating a focus on specific nutrients to maintain general health and well-being. The following are key nutrients and their food sources that are particularly important for seniors;

I.   **Protein**: Protein is essential for sustaining muscular mass, strength, and overall bodily function.
Sources: Lean meats (chicken, turkey, and fish), eggs, dairy products (milk, yogurt, and cheese), legumes (beans and lentils), nuts, seeds, and tofu.

II.   **Calcium**: Calcium is essential for bone health, preventing osteoporosis and fractures.
Sources: Dairy items (milk, cheese,

yogurt), fortified plant-based milk alternatives (soy milk, almond milk), leafy green vegetables (kale, collard greens), canned bone-in fish (sardines, salmon), and calcium-enriched meals (orange juice, cereal).

III. **Vitamin D**: Vitamin D helps bone health and immunological function and may lower the risk of falls.

Sources: sunlight exposure (restricted for older people), fatty fish (salmon, mackerel, tuna), egg yolks, fortified meals (milk, cereal, orange juice), and supplements as needed.

IV. **Vitamin B12**: Vitamin B12 is essential for neuron function, red blood cell synthesis, and energy metabolism.

Sources: Animal goods (meat, fish, poultry, eggs, dairy), fortified foods (cereals, plant-based milk replacements), and supplements for people who have difficulty absorbing nutrients.

V. **Fiber**: Fiber promotes digestive health, prevents constipation, and may lower the risk of heart disease and type 2 diabetes. **Sources**: Whole grains (oatmeal, brown rice, quinoa), fruits (apples, berries, oranges), vegetables (broccoli, Brussels sprouts, carrots), legumes (beans, lentils), nuts, and seeds.

VI. **Potassium**: Important for maintaining appropriate blood pressure, heart function, and muscle contractions.
Sources: Fruits (bananas, oranges, apricots), vegetables (potatoes, sweet potatoes, tomatoes), dairy products, fish, chicken, and beans.

VII. **Omega-3 Fatty Acids**: Promotes heart health, brain function, and inflammation reduction.
Sources: fatty fish (salmon, mackerel, and trout), flaxseeds, chia seeds, walnuts, and omega-3-enriched eggs.

VIII. **Antioxidants (vitamin C, vitamin E, and selenium)**: They help prevent cells from free radical damage, may lessen the incidence of chronic illnesses, and boost immunological function.

Sources: Fruits (citrus, berries, and kiwi), vegetables (bell peppers, spinach, and broccoli), nuts, seeds, whole grains, and lean meats are all good sources.

IX. **Fluids (water)**: Important for hydration, digestion, temperature regulation, and overall health.

Sources: Include water, herbal teas, broth-based soups, fruits, vegetables, and diluted fruit juices.

Macronutrient Balance for Optimal Health

Balancing macronutrients is crucial for overall health, as they provide the body with energy and important nutrients for numerous bodily activities. Here's how you can get a balanced macronutrient intake:

Carbohydrates

- **Role**: Primary source of energy for the body, especially for cognitive function and physical activity.

- **Healthy Sources**: Whole grains (brown rice, quinoa, and oats), fruits, vegetables, legumes (beans and lentils), and starchy veggies (sweet potatoes and squash) are all good sources.
- **Balancing Tip**: Choose complex carbohydrates over refined carbohydrates for long-lasting energy and important nutrients like fiber, vitamins, and minerals.

Protein

- **Role**: Protein plays a vital role in tissue healing, immunological function, and enzyme and hormone production.
- **Healthy Sources**: Lean meats (chicken, turkey, and fish), eggs, dairy products (milk, yogurt, and cheese), legumes (beans and lentils), nuts, seeds, and tofu are all good sources of nutrition.
- **Balancing Tip**: Include protein in each meal and snack to enhance satiety, muscle maintenance, and overall health.

Fat

- **Role**: Provides energy, promotes cell structure, absorbs fat-soluble vitamins (A, D, E, and K), and aids in hormone production.
- **Healthy Sources**: Avocados, nuts, seeds, olive oil, avocado oil, and fatty fish (trout, mackerel, and salmon) are good sources of unsaturated fats.
- **Balancing Tip**: Aim to consume a range of healthy fats while reducing saturated and trans fats found in processed meals, fried foods, and baked products.

Balancing Tips

- **Portion Control**: Pay attention to portion sizes and strive for a balanced macronutrient distribution at each meal.
- **Prioritize Whole Foods**: To increase nutritional intake and boost overall wellness, choose nutrient-dense, whole foods over processed and refined items.

- **Listen to Your Body**: Pay attention to hunger and fullness cues and alter your macronutrient intake to fit your body's requirements.
- **Meal Planning**: Plan meals and snacks that include a variety of carbohydrates, protein, and healthy fats to help you stay energized and healthy throughout the day.
- **Stay Hydrated**: Drink lots of water throughout the day to help with digestion, vitamin absorption, and overall hydration, which can affect energy levels and hunger control.

Hydration: An Ofen-Overlooked Phenomenon

Hydration is an important but often overlooked aspect of general health and well-being. Here's why staying hydrated is essential and how to ensure enough hydration:

Importance of Hydration

1. **Regulates Body Temperature**: Water helps control body temperature by sweating and evaporation, which is especially important during hot weather or physical activity.

2. **Promotes Digestion and Nutrient Absorption**: Adequate hydration aids in the digestion and absorption of nutrients from food, allowing the body to use nutrients more efficiently.

3. **Flushes Toxins**: Water aids in the elimination of waste products and toxins from the body via urine, perspiration, and bowel movements, thereby promoting kidney function and detoxification.

4. **Maintains Blood Volume and Pressure**: Staying hydrated helps keep blood volume and pressure in healthy ranges, which supports cardiovascular health and circulation.

5. **Promotes Joint Health**: Water lubricates and cushions joints, reducing friction and discomfort, which is especially useful for

individuals who have arthritis or joint problems.

Tips for Maintaining Adequate Hydration

a. **Drink Plenty of Water**: Aim to drink at least 8–10 glasses (64–80 ounces) of water each day, or more if you're physically active or live in a hot region.

b. **Monitor Urine Color**: Check the color of your urine; pale yellow to clear suggests adequate hydration, but dark yellow or amber may indicate dehydration.

c. **Consume Hydrating Foods**: Include hydrating foods with high water content in your diet, such as fruits (watermelon, strawberries, and oranges), vegetables (cucumbers, tomatoes, and celery), soups, and broths.

d. **Sip Throughout the Day**: Rather than waiting until you're thirsty, drink water frequently throughout the day to stay hydrated.

e. **Limit Dehydrating Beverages**: Avoid drinking caffeinated and alcoholic beverages, since they can increase urine production and lead to dehydration.

f. **Set Reminders**: Use alarms or smartphone apps to remind yourself to drink water regularly, especially if you are prone to forgetting.

g. **Hydrate Before and After Exercise**: Drink water before, during, and after exercise to replenish fluids lost through perspiration and avoid dehydration.

Chapter 3: Senior-Safe Exercise

The Importance of Exercise in Weight Loss and Muscle Preservation.

Exercise is important for both weight loss and muscle preservation, especially as individuals age. Here's how exercise helps with these goals:

Weight Loss

- **Calorie Expenditure**: Exercise raises calorie expenditure, which contributes to the calorie deficit required for weight loss. Regular exercise, combined with a well-balanced diet, promotes fat loss while maintaining lean muscle mass.
- **Metabolic Rate**: Regular physical activity increases metabolism, even at rest, which can help with weight loss by increasing calorie burn throughout the day.
- **Appetite Regulation**: Exercise regulates appetite hormones, resulting in improved control of food intake and fewer cravings

for harmful foods, which aids in weight loss attempts.

- **Fat Loss vs. Muscle Loss**: Incorporating aerobic (cardio) and resistance (strength) training in an exercise plan increases fat reduction while maintaining lean muscle mass, resulting in a healthy body composition.

Muscle Preservation

- **Resistance Training**: Strength training techniques, such as lifting weights or utilizing resistance bands, promote muscular development and maintenance. This is especially significant for older adults, who are prone to age-related muscle loss (sarcopenia).
- **Bone Health**: Weight-bearing exercises, such as resistance training, help to maintain bone density and strength, which reduces the risk of osteoporosis and fracture.
- **Functional Fitness**: Strong muscles enable greater balance, coordination, and

mobility, minimizing the risk of falls and injuries, which can be particularly useful for older adults.

- **Metabolic Health**: Lean muscle mass is important for metabolic health because it increases resting metabolic rate (RMR) and improves insulin sensitivity, which helps manage blood sugar levels and reduces the risk of metabolic illnesses like type 2 diabetes.

- **Overall Well-Being**: Regular exercise increases mental health, reduces stress, and improves sleep quality, all of which contribute to overall well-being and quality of life, especially as individuals age.

Tip for Effective Exercise

1. **Combination Approach**: Include both aerobic and resistance training workouts in your regimen for maximum results.

2. **Progressive Overload**: Gradually increase the intensity, duration, or resistance of your workouts over time to

keep your muscles challenged and adapting.

3. **Consistency**: Aim for at least 150 minutes of moderate-intensity aerobic activity or 75 minutes of vigorous-intensity aerobic activity per week, along with two or more days of strength training.

4. **Variety**: Keep your workouts interesting and pleasurable by experimenting with different sorts of exercises and activities that target different muscle groups and prevent monotony.

5. **Listen to Your Body**: Pay attention to your body's signals and modify your training regimen as needed to avoid injury and encourage healing.

Recommended Exercise Types: Cardio, Strength Training, Flexibility, and Balance

To obtain a well-rounded fitness regimen that promotes general health and well-being, incorporate a variety of exercise styles, such as cardio, strength training, flexibility, and balancing activities. Here's a breakdown of each type, with recommended activities within each category:

1. **Cardiovascular Exercise (Cardio)**

Goals: increase endurance, improve heart health, burn calories, and improve mood.

Recommend Activities:

Pace walking vigorously

Jogging or running

Cycling

Swimming

Dancing

Aerobic classes (such as step aerobics and Zumba)

Elliptical training

Rolling

2. **Strength Training**

Goals: Promote muscle strength and mass, boost metabolism, increase bone density, and support functional motions.

Recommended Activities:

Weightlifting (using dumbbells, barbells, or resistance bands)

bodyweight exercises (push-ups, squats, lunges, and planks)

Weight machines at the gym

Functional training exercises (e.g., kettlebell swings and medicine ball workouts)

Pilates

3. Flexibility Training

Goal: Aim to develop a range of motion, reduce muscle tension, avoid injuries, and improve posture.

Recommended Activities:

Stretching exercises, either static or dynamic.

Yoga

Pilates

Tai Chi

Foam rolling or self-myofascial release

4. Balance exercises:

Goals: Improves stability, coordination, and proprioception (awareness of body position in space), which reduces the chance of falling.

Recommended Activities:

Standing on one leg (with support if needed)

Tandem walk (heel-to-toe).

Balancing with a stability ball or balance board.

Tai Chi

Yoga poses that challenge balance (e.g., tree pose and warrior III)

Balance-focused group fitness classes

Tips for Incorporating Exercise

I. **Variety**: Aim for a well-balanced mix of cardio, strength, flexibility, and balance exercises to target various parts of fitness and avoid monotony.

II. **Progression**: Gradually increase the intensity, duration, or complexity of your workouts over time to keep your body challenged and progressing.

III. **Consistency**: Schedule frequent exercise sessions throughout the week, aiming for at least 150 minutes of moderate-intensity aerobic activity or 75 minutes of vigorous-intensity aerobic activity, as well as two or more days of strength training per week.

IV. **Safety**: Prioritize appropriate form and technique to avoid injuries, and pay attention to your body's signals. Before beginning a new exercise program, consult with a healthcare provider or a fitness professional, especially if you have any underlying health conditions or concerns.

Setting Realistic and Safe Workout Goals

Setting realistic and safe workout goals is essential for making progress while reducing the risk of injury and burnout. Here are some guidelines for developing attainable goals:

1. Start Slowly and Gradually

Tips: Begin with manageable activities, gradually increasing intensity, duration, or frequency over time.

Example: Start with short walks or low-resistance workouts, then gradually increase the distance, pace, or resistance as your fitness improves.

2. Be Specific and Measurable

Tip: Define your goals clearly and create measurable criteria for tracking success.

Example: Instead of striving to "get in shape," set a goal like walking 30 minutes three times a week or completing a particular number of strength training sessions per week.

3. Consider Your Current Fitness Level

Tips: Set goals that are both challenging and attainable based on your current fitness level, health status, and lifestyle.

Example: If you're new to fitness, start with beginner-friendly activities and work your way up as you build strength, endurance, and confidence.

4. Prioritize Behavior Improvements

Tip: Prioritize developing healthy habits and lifestyle improvements above focusing exclusively on weight loss or muscle gain.

Example: Set consistent goals, such as sticking to a regular workout routine or exploring new sorts of physical activity.

5. Divide Goals into Smaller Milestones

Tips: Break down huge goals into smaller, achievable milestones to maintain motivation and celebrate your accomplishments along the way.

Example: If your ultimate goal is to run a 5K, begin by walking or running for 1 mile without stopping, then progressively increase the distance and pace.

6. Be Flexible and Realistic

Tips: Assign challenging yet realistic goals, considering factors such as time restraints, physical restrictions, and other obligations.

Example: Instead of attempting to exercise every day, choose a more realistic target of three to four times per week, with the flexibility to change depending on your schedule and energy levels.

7. Listen to Your Body

Tip: Modify your goals and activities according to your body's signals to avoid overexertion and injury.

Example: If you're feeling fatigued or uncomfortable, consider taking a rest day or modifying your workout intensity.

8. Seek Support and Accountability

Tips: Share your goals with friends, family, or a gym buddy to stay accountable and encouraged.

Example: Join a fitness class, hire a personal trainer, or join online communities to meet people who have similar goals and experiences.

Chapter 4: Developing Healthy Eating Habits

How to Create a Balanced Meal Plan

A balanced meal plan consists of integrating a range of nutrient-rich foods from various food groups to ensure that you achieve your nutritional requirements while also maintaining your overall health. Here's a step-by-step guide for creating a balanced meal plan:

Determine Your Calorie Needs:

- Calculate your daily calorie requirements based on age, gender, weight, height, exercise level, and weight goals.
- For personalized guidance, use an online calculator or consult a healthcare provider or registered dietitian.

Choose Nutrient-Dense Foods:

- Focus on incorporating a variety of nutrient-dense foods in your meal, like

fruits, vegetables, whole grains, lean proteins, and healthy fats.
- Consume fewer processed and refined foods, sugary snacks, and high-fat, high-calorie items.

Split Plate:

- Utilize the dish strategy to visibly split your dish into sections.
- Fill half of your plate with non-starchy vegetables (e.g., leafy greens, broccoli, and bell peppers).
- Reserve a quarter of your plate for lean proteins (e.g., chicken, fish, tofu, and beans).
- Allocate the remaining quarter for whole grains or starchy vegetables (such as brown rice, quinoa, and sweet potatoes).

Include a Variety of Foods:

- Choose various fruits, vegetables, grains, and proteins to add a diversity of hues, flavors, and textures to your meals.

- To ensure you obtain a range of nutrients and avoid dietary boredom, rotate your food choices.

Balance Macronutrients:

- Include carbohydrates, proteins, and healthy fats in each meal for sustained energy, to promote satiety, and to support general health.
- Choose complex carbs (whole grains, legumes), lean proteins (poultry, fish, eggs), and unsaturated fats (avocado, olive oil, nuts).

Pay Attention to Portion Sizes:

- Eat in moderation to prevent overeating and maintain a balanced diet.
- Use measuring cups, spoons, or visual cues to determine the proper serving sizes for various food groups.

Plan and Prep:

- Plan your weekly meals based on your schedule, preferences, and nutritional goals.
- Streamline meal preparation easier during the week; prepare ingredients in advance, such as washing and cutting vegetables, cooking grains and proteins, and portioning out snacks.

Listen to Your Body:

- Pay attention to hunger and fullness cues, and eat consciously to prevent overeating or undereating.
- Adjust your meal plan as needed to reflect your energy levels, cravings, and dietary preferences.

Stay Hydrated:

- Include fluids in your balanced meal plan, such as water, herbal teas, low-fat milk, or plant-based milk alternatives.

Understanding Portion Proportions and Meal Timing

Understanding portion proportions and meal scheduling is essential for maintaining a balanced and nutritious diet. Here's a handy guide to navigating portion sizes and meal timing:

Portion Size:

- **Vegetables**: Try to fill half of your plate with non-starchy veggies such as leafy greens, broccoli, carrots, and bell peppers. A normal serving size is one cup of raw veggies or half a cup of cooked vegetables.
- **Protein**: Include a palm-sized serving of lean protein, such as chicken, fish, tofu, beans, or lentils, in your meal. A serving size is typically 3–4 ounces, or about the size of a deck of cards.
- **Grains/Starches**: Choose whole grains or starchy vegetables like brown rice, quinoa, sweet potatoes, or whole grain bread. A serving size is usually about 1/2 cup of cooked grains or 1 slice of bread.

- **Fats**: Incorporate healthy fats like avocado, nuts, seeds, and olive oil into your meals in moderation. A serving size for fats is usually 1-2 teaspoons or a small handful.
- **Fruits**: Include a serving of fruit with each meal or as a snack. A serving size is usually one medium-sized fruit (e.g., apple, banana) or 1/2 cup chopped fruit.

Meal Timing:

- **Breakfast**: Eat a healthy breakfast within an hour or two of waking up to jumpstart your metabolism and provide you with energy for the day ahead. Include a variety of carbohydrates, proteins, and fats to keep you satisfied and stimulated.
- **Lunch**: Have a midday meal that consists of lean protein, whole grains, vegetables, and healthy fats. Aim to eat lunch roughly 4-5 hours after breakfast to maintain consistent energy levels throughout the day.

- **Dinner**: Have a well-rounded dinner with similar components to lunch, concentrating on portion sizes and nutrient balance. Try to eat dinner at least 2–3 hours before bedtime to allow for digestion and improve sleep quality.
- **Snacks**: Include nutritious snacks in between meals to satisfy hunger and avoid overeating at mealtime. Choose nutrient-dense options such as fruit and nut butter, Greek yogurt with berries, or raw vegetables with hummus.
- **Hydration**: Drink water throughout the day and with each meal to stay hydrated. Aim to drink at least 8 glasses (64 ounces) of water every day, adjusting based on activity level and personal hydration requirements.

Tips on Portion Control and Meal Timing

I. **Use Visual Cues**: Use everyday objects or your hand size to determine portion proportions (e.g., a fist for grains, and a palm for protein).

II.   **Practice Mindful Eating**: pay attention to hunger and fullness cues, and eat gently to savor your food and avoid overeating.

III.   **Plan**: Plan your meals and snacks ahead of time to ensure proper nutrition and avoid impulsive food choices.

IV.   **Listen to Your Body**: Eat when you're starving and quit when you're satisfied, rather than eating according to a strict schedule.

V.   **Stay Consistent**: Aim to eat meals and snacks at similar times each day to control hunger and preserve energy levels.

Tips for Mindful Eating and Managing Cravings

Mindful eating and regulating cravings can help you develop a healthier connection with food, create healthier food choices, and maintain a nutritious diet. Here are some tips to help you incorporate mindful eating and effectively manage cravings:

Mindful Eating

- **Eat Without Distractions**: To focus on the sensory experience of eating, turn off TV, smartphones, and computers.

- **Chew Slowly**: Take your time chewing each bite fully and enjoying the flavors, textures, and aromas of your food.

- **Pay Attention to Hunger Cues**: Listen to your body's famine and fullness cues, eating when you're famished and quitting when you're satisfied, instead of eating out of habit or emotion.

- **Practice Gratitude**: Before eating, take a moment to express gratitude for the meals in front of you and the nourishment they provide to your body.

- **Use All Five Senses**: While eating, pay attention to the colors, flavors, tastes, textures, and sounds of your meal.

- **Eat Mindfully:** Be present and nonjudgmental throughout meals, observing thoughts and emotions without labeling or criticizing.

Managing Cravings

- **Identify Triggers**: Recognize the factors that cause cravings, such as stress, boredom, or certain food cues.
- **Find Healthy Substitutes**: Replace unhealthy cravings with healthier alternatives that satisfy your cravings while also supplying nutrients, such as fruit instead of candy or air-popped popcorn in place of chips.
- **Practice Moderation**: Allow yourself to consume moderate portions of your favorite foods occasionally, rather than starving yourself completely, to avoid feelings of deprivation and overeating later.
- **Stay Hydrated**: Drink water throughout the day, as thirst can be misinterpreted as hunger, resulting in unnecessary cravings.
- **Manage Stress**: Find healthy ways to cope with stress, such as exercise, meditation, deep breathing, or spending time in nature, to reduce emotional eating and stress-induced cravings.

- **Plan Ahead**: Plan your meals and snacks ahead of time, including healthy options that you enjoy, to avoid making impulsive decisions and craving unhealthy foods.

Chapter 5: Overcoming Weight Loss Challenges

Addressing Frequent Challenges to Weight Loss After 60

Addressing frequent weight loss challenges after the age of 60 demands a holistic approach that takes into account both physical and lifestyle issues. Here are some frequent challenges and how to overcome them:

Slower Metabolism

- **Barrier**: Metabolism tends to slow down with age, making weight loss more tough.
- **Strategy**: Increase physical activity to burn more calories and retain muscle mass, which can help compensate for a slower metabolism. Incorporate strength-training workouts to build muscle and increase metabolism.

Hormonal Changes

- **Barrier**: Lowered estrogen and testosterone levels can impact metabolism and body composition.
- **Strategy**: Consult a healthcare professional about hormone replacement therapy or other medical procedures, if necessary. Maintain a balanced diet and a regular exercise routine to support overall health and weight management.

Sarcopenia (muscle loss)

- **Barrier**: Age-related muscle loss (sarcopenia) can impair metabolism and physical function in older persons.
- **Strategy**: Include strength training activities in your workout routine to help you build and maintain muscle mass. Squats, lunges, push-ups, and resistance band workouts are excellent options for targeting all main muscle groups.

Joint Pain and Mobility Issues

- **Barrier**: Joint discomfort, arthritis, or mobility difficulties can restrict physical activity and make exercise difficult.
- **Strategy**: Swimming, cycling, walking, or water aerobics are examples of low-impact, joint-friendly exercises. Consider consulting with a physical therapist or personal trainer to develop a tailored fitness regimen that meets your requirements and skills.

Medications

- **Barrier**: Some medications might induce weight gain or make weight loss more difficult.
- **Strategy**: Talk to your healthcare provider about the possible side effects of your medications and talk about choices if weight gain is a concern. Focus on healthy lifestyle practices, including a balanced diet and regular exercise, to manage weight despite medication use.

Emotional Eating and Stress

- **Barrier**: Emotional eating and stress can lead to overeating and ruin weight loss efforts.
- **Strategy**: Deep breathing, meditation, yoga, or spending time in nature can all help to reduce stress and emotional eating. While emotional eating is preventing you from losing weight, seek support from friends, family, or a therapist.

Social and Environmental

- **Barriers**: Eating habits can be influenced by social events, family gatherings, and environmental cues, making it challenging to stick to a balanced diet.
- **Strategy**: Prepare for social gatherings by choosing healthier options, practicing portion control, and focusing on mindful eating. Surround yourself with supportive friends and family members who promote healthy habits and value your dietary preferences.

Slow Progress and Plateaus

- **Barrier**: Weight loss progress may stall or stagnate as you age, leading to frustration and discouragement.
- **Strategy**: Concentrate on non-scale victories such as enhanced energy, sleep quality, or increased strength and mobility. Be patient and consistent in your healthy practices, and remember that delayed progress is still progress.

Lack of Motivation

- **Barrier**: Perceived impediments can prevent people from sticking to their weight loss goal.
- **Strategy**: Set reasonable and achievable goals, celebrate small successes along the way, and engage in activities that you enjoy and that make you feel good. Enlist the support of a friend, family member, or health coach to help you stay accountable and motivated.

How to Stay Motivated and Track Progress

Staying motivated and tracking progress are key components of establishing and maintaining success in any health or fitness journey. Here are some techniques to help you stay motivated and properly track your progress:

Staying Motivated

- **Set Clear Goals**: Establish specific, measurable, achievable, relevant, and time-bound (SMART) goals to provide a clear direction and purpose for your trip.
- **Discover Your Why**: Determine your intrinsic motives and reasons for wanting to achieve your objectives. Connecting with your deepest motivations, whether it's to improve your health, increase your energy level, or set a good example for loved ones, can fuel your determination.
- **Visualize Success**: Use visualization techniques to envision yourself reaching your objectives and reaping the advantages of your efforts. Visualizing achievement can boost motivation and reinforce beneficial habits.

- **Break It Down**: Break down your goals into smaller, more doable activities or milestones to avoid overwhelm and celebrate your progress.
- **Maintain a Positive Mindset**: Focus on your strengths, progress, and successes rather than dwelling on setbacks or obstacles. Develop self-compassion and treat yourself with care and understanding.
- **Surround Yourself With Support**: Seek encouragement and support from friends, family, or a supportive group of people who share similar aims and values.
- **Reward Yourself**: Celebrate your accomplishments and milestones with non-food rewards like a relaxing bath, new workout outfits, or a fun outing with friends.

Tracking Progress

- **Keep a Journal**: Record your daily activities, workouts, food, thoughts, and emotions in a journal or digital tracker. Tracking progress enables you to detect patterns, monitor changes over time, and adapt your strategy as necessary.

- **Use Apps or Technology**: Utilize fitness apps, wearable devices, or internet trackers to track your physical activity, nutrition, sleep, and other health-related metrics. These tools can provide useful data and insights to keep you on track.

- **Measure Your Progress**: Take regular measurements of your progress, such as body weight, body measurements, body fat percentage, and fitness tests. Tracking your actual achievements can help motivate and validate your efforts.

- **Create Accountability**: Share your goals and progress with an accountability partner, coach, or mentor who can offer support, encouragement, and accountability along the way.

- **Reflect and Adjust**: Review your progress regularly and reflect on what is working well and what areas may need to be adjusted. Be willing to adjust your plan based on your observations and feedback.

- **Celebrate Milestones**: acknowledge and celebrate your accomplishments, no matter how small, to stay motivated and reinforce positive behaviors.

Managing Plateaus and Maintaining Weight Reduction

Dealing with plateaus and maintaining weight reduction requires patience, persistence, and a proactive approach to overcome challenges. Here are some techniques for overcoming plateaus and maintaining your weight loss progress:

Dealing with Plateaus

- **Reassess Your Habits**: Examine your diet, exercise routine, sleep patterns, stress levels, and other lifestyle factors to identify areas that may require change.
- **Mix Up Your Exercises**: Add variation to your exercise regimen by attempting new activities, changing the intensity or duration of your exercises, or

incorporating different forms of training (for example, strength training, cardio, and flexibility).

- **Adjust Your Caloric Consumption**: If you've been following a calorie-restricted diet, reassess your caloric requirements and adjust your consumption accordingly. To stimulate further progress, gradually reduce portion sizes or make minor adjustments to your macronutrient ratios.

- **Focus on Strength Training**: Increase the intensity and frequency of your strength training workouts to build muscle mass and enhance metabolism. Muscle burns more calories at rest than fat, so increasing muscle mass can help you get beyond plateaus.

- **Monitor Your Progress**: Keep track of your food intake, activity, and other important metrics regularly to discover any potential hazards or tendencies that may be contributing to the plateau.

- **Stay Hydrated**: Drink enough water throughout the day, as dehydration can mimic hunger and contribute to overeating.

- **Manage Stress**: To reduce stress, practice stress-management techniques such as mindfulness, meditation, deep breathing exercises, or yoga, as high cortisol levels might interfere with weight loss efforts.
- **Get Enough Sleep**: Aim for 7-9 hours of quality sleep per night, as insufficient sleep can disturb hormonal balance, increase appetite, and affect metabolism.

Maintaining Weight Loss

- **Establish Healthy Habits**: Concentrate on developing long-term behaviors that improve general health and well-being, such as eating a balanced diet, being active, getting adequate sleep, managing stress, and staying hydrated.
- **Monitor Your Eating Patterns**: Keep an eye on your hunger and fullness clues, practice portion control, and steer clear of mindless or emotional eating habits.

- **Stay Active**: Make physical activity a regular part of your day by selecting activities you enjoy and adding them to your routine. Aim for 150 minutes of moderate-intensity aerobic activity or 75 minutes of vigorous-intensity aerobic activity per week, along with strength training exercises at least two days per week.

- **Be Aware of Trigger Foods**: Determine which foods or settings may contribute to overeating or unhealthy choices, and develop techniques to manage cravings and navigate challenging situations.

- **Practice Self-Conpassion**: Be kind to yourself and avoid harsh self-criticism or guilt if you indulge or have setbacks on occasion. Remember that losing weight is a long-term process, and it's common to encounter setbacks along the way.

Seek Support

- **Create a Support Network**: Surround yourself with friends, family, or a supportive community that can offer encouragement, accountability, and understanding as you embark on your weight reduction journey.

- **Seek Professional Help**: If you're struggling to overcome plateaus or maintain weight reduction on your own, try consulting with a registered dietitian, personal trainer, or therapist who can offer specific recommendations and support.

Chapter 6: Recipes and Meal Ideas

Simple, Healthy Recipes Tailored to Older Adults

As we age, we must nourish our bodies with healthy foods that promote general health and well-being. In this chapter, we'll look at simple and delicious recipes for older individuals, with an emphasis on nutrient-dense ingredients and easy-to-prepare meals that promote vitality and longevity.

Breakfast Options

Overnight Oats with Berries and Nuts

Ingredients:

- 1/2 cup rolled oats
- 1/2 cup unsweetened almond milk (or other milk of choice).
- 1/4 cup Greek yogurt.
- 1/2 cup mixed berries (such as strawberries, blueberries, and raspberries).

- 1 tablespoon chopped nuts (such as almonds and walnuts)
- Optional: sprinkle with honey or maple syrup.

Instructions:

- In a jar or bowl, combine the rolled oats, almond milk, and Greek yogurt. Stir well to mix.
- Place the mixed berries and chopped nuts on top.
- Cover and refrigerate overnight.
- In the morning, stir it and serve it cold or warm.

Veggie Omelet

Ingredients

- 2 eggs
- 1/4 cup of diced bell pepper
- 1/4 cup chopped tomatoes
- 1/4 cup chopped spinach
- Salt and pepper to taste.
- 1 tablespoon of olive oil

Instructions:

- Whisk eggs in a bowl until thoroughly mixed. Season with salt and pepper.
- In a nonstick skillet set over medium heat, warm the olive oil.
- Add the diced bell peppers, tomatoes, and spinach to the skillet. Cook for 2–3 minutes, until the vegetables have slightly softened.
- Pour the whisked eggs over the vegetables and turn the skillet to spread them evenly.
- Cook for 2–3 minutes, until the bottom set. Carefully flip the omelet and cook for an additional 1-2 minutes until fully done.
- Serve hot with whole-grain bread or fruit.

Lunch and Dinner Ideas

Quinoa Salad with Chickpeas and Roasted Vegetables

Ingredients:

- 1/2 cup cooked quinoa

- 1/2 cup cooked chickpeas (canned, rinsed, and drained).
- 1 cup mixed roasted veggies (such as bell peppers, zucchini, and eggplant)
- Handful of fresh spinach leaves.
- Lemon-tahini dressing (1 tablespoon tahini, juice of 1/2 lemon,
- 1 teaspoon olive oil
- Salt, and pepper to taste.

Instructions:

- In a bowl, combine cooked quinoa, chickpeas, roasted veggies, and spinach leaves.
- Drizzle with lemon-tahini dressing and toss to coat.
- Serve as a hearty salad or as a side dish for grilled chicken or fish.

Baked Salmon with Lemon and Herbs

Ingredients:

- 1 salmon fillet (4-6 ounces)
- 1 tablespoon of olive oil.

- 1/2 lemon juice
- 1 teaspoon dried herbs, such as dill, thyme, and rosemary
- Season with salt and pepper to taste.

Instructions:

- Preheat the oven to 400°F (200°C). Cover a baking sheet with parchment paper.
- Arrange the salmon fillet on a baking pan. Drizzle the dish with olive oil and lemon juice.
- Sprinkle with dried herbs, salt, and pepper.
- Bake for 12–15 minutes, or until the salmon is thoroughly cooked and readily flaked with a fork.
- Serve hot with steamed vegetables or a salad.

Snacks and Dessert Options

Greek Yogurt with Honey and Almonds

Ingredients:

- 1/2 cup Greek yogurt.
- 1 tablespoon of honey
- 1 tablespoon chopped almonds.

Instructions:

- Place Greek yogurt in a bowl.
- Drizzle with honey, and sprinkle with chopped almonds.
- Enjoy it as a filling snack or light dessert.

Fruit Salad with Mint Lime Dressing

Ingredients:

- Seasonal fruits (such as melon, berries, grapes, and kiwi)
- 1 lime juice
- 1 tablespoon chopped fresh mint leaves.
- Optional: sprinkle with honey or maple syrup.

Instructions:

- Cut the various fruits into bite-sized pieces and place them in a bowl.

- In a small mixing bowl, combine lime juice, chopped mint leaves, and optional honey or maple syrup.
- Pour the dressing over the fruit salad and toss to combine.
- For optimal flavor, refrigerate for half an hour before serving.

These simple and healthy meals are designed to fulfill the dietary demands of older people, supplying important nutrients while also appealing to their taste buds. Experiment with these recipes and tailor them to your specific preferences and dietary needs for delicious meals that promote your health and well-being.

Meal Planning Ideas and Healthy Snack Suggestions

Meal planning and smart snacking are essential components of eating a nutritious diet and staying healthy. Here are some meal-planning ideas and suggestions for healthy snacking:

Meal Planning Tips:

Plan Balanced Meals: To ensure a healthy diet, incorporate a variety of food groups into each meal, such as lean proteins, whole grains, fruits, vegetables, and healthy fats.

Batch Cooking: Prepare larger batches of meals and portion them into individual servings for use throughout the week. This can save time and make it easier to maintain a balanced eating routine.

Add Variety: Experiment with new recipes, cuisines, and flavors to keep meals interesting and minimize boredom. For a pleasurable dining experience, use a variety of colors, textures, and flavors.

Creatively Repurpose Leftovers: For quick and convenient meals, repurpose leftovers into salads, soups, sandwiches, or wraps.

Plan Snacks: Incorporate nutritious snacks into your meal plan to help manage hunger between meals and avoid unhealthful food choices. Choose nutrient-dense foods such as fresh fruit, raw veggies with hummus, Greek yogurt, nuts and seeds, or whole-grain crackers with cheese.

Consider Dietary Preferences and Limits: When planning meals, take into account any dietary preferences, allergies, or limits to ensure that everyone's needs are fulfilled. Consider alternate ingredients and substitutions as needed.

Tips for Healthy Snacking

Choose Nutrient-Dense Foods: Look for snacks that are high in important nutrients and energy but low in calories, sugar, and bad fats. Choose entire foods such as fruits, vegetables, nuts, seeds, yogurt, and whole-grain snacks.

Portion Control: While snacking, be conscious of your portion amounts to avoid overeating. Portion snacks into small bowls or containers and avoid mindlessly eating from huge packets.

Plan Ahead: Prepare healthy snacks ahead of time and portion them into grab-and-go containers or bags for convenient access throughout the day. Keep pre-cut fruits and veggies, trail mix, or yogurt cups in the refrigerator for quick and easy snacking.

Stay Hydrated: Thirst might be confused with appetite. Drink water throughout the day and choose hydrating snacks like fresh fruits and vegetables.

Listen to Your Body: Pay attention to your hunger and fullness cues, and snack when you're hungry, not out of boredom or habit. Choose snacks that will fulfill your cravings while also providing you with long-lasting energy.

Mindful Eating: Savor each bite, eat slowly, and focus on the flavors, textures, and feelings of the meal. To truly enjoy and appreciate your food, avoid distractions such as television or screens while snacking.

By adopting these meal planning ideas and healthy snacking suggestions into your daily routine, you can make more informed food choices, meet your nutritional needs, and live a healthier life. Remember, consistency and balance are key to long-term success in sustaining healthy eating habits.

Adapting Favorite Recipes to Be Healthy

Adapting favorite recipes to make them healthier is a great way to eat your favorite foods while also benefiting your health and wellness. Here are some suggestions for making healthier alternatives and modifications to recipes.

1. Reduce Added Sugar

Replace Sugar with Natural Sweeteners: Instead of refined sugar, use natural sweeteners such as honey, maple syrup, or mashed ripe bananas in recipes.

Use Less Sweetener: Reduce the amount of sugar or sweetener used in recipes gradually as your taste buds adjust over time.

2. Increase Fiber

Choose Whole Grains: Instead of refined grains, use whole grains like whole wheat flour, brown rice, quinoa, or oats.

Add Fiber-Rich Ingredients: Incorporate fiber-rich items such as beans, lentils, vegetables, fruits, nuts, and seeds into soups, salads, casseroles, and stir-fry recipes.

3. Reduce Saturated Fat

Choose Leaner Proteins: Select lean cuts of meat, skinless chicken, and fish instead of higher-fat options. Alternatively, use plant-based protein bases like beans, tofu, tempeh, or legumes in recipes.

Use Healthier Cooking Techniques: To cut down on extra fat and calories, bake, grill, steam, or roast instead of frying.

4. Increase Nutrient Density

Increase Veggies: Incorporate a range of colorful veggies into your dishes to improve vitamins, minerals, and antioxidants. Consider adding more vegetables to soups, stews, pasta, and casseroles.

Include Leafy Greens: Leafy greens such as spinach, kale, or Swiss chard can be added to smoothies, omelets, stir-fries, and salads to boost their nutritional value.

5. Reduce Sodium

Use Herbs and Spices: Instead of using salt to season foods, use herbs, spices, and citrus zest. Experiment with various flavor combinations to improve the taste of your favorite recipes.

Choose Low-Sodium Ingredients. Choose low-sodium or no-salt canned items such as beans, tomatoes, and broth, and restrict the use of high-sodium condiments such as soy sauce and Worcestershire sauce.

6. Control Portion Size

Portion Control: When serving meals and snacks, consider the size of the servings. Use smaller dishes, bowls, and utensils to help regulate portion sizes and avoid overeating.

Focus on Balanced Meals. To increase satiety and avoid excess calorie consumption, aim for a mix of protein, carbs, and healthy fats in each meal.

7. Modify Cooking Techniques

Trim Excess Fat: Before cooking, remove any visible fat from meat and poultry to reduce saturated fat intake.

-Skim Fat from Soups and Stews: Refrigerate soups and stews before serving to firm the fat, then remove the hardened fat layer from the surface before reheating and serving.

8. Enhance Flavor Without Adding Calories

Experiment with Flavorful Ingredients: To add flavor to recipes without adding calories or unhealthy fats, try using garlic, onions, ginger, fresh herbs, citrus juice, vinegar, and mustard.

Conclusion

As we wrap up "Healthy Weight Loss After 60: A Guide to Vitality and Longevity," it's important to reflect on the transforming discoveries and empowering solutions we've discovered together. Throughout this guide, we've looked at the specific obstacles and opportunities that come with losing weight in our golden years, as well as practical skills and knowledge to support your path towards a healthier, happier self.

Now armed with knowledge, inspiration, and a renewed sense of purpose, it's time to take action and make the required changes to achieve your health and weight reduction goals. Remember that growth is not always linear, and setbacks might occur along the way. However, with patience, perseverance, and a dedication to self-care, you can overcome challenges and achieve long-term success.

As you begin this new chapter in your health journey, remember to be kind to yourself and celebrate every triumph, no matter how small. Surround yourself with positive people who uplift and inspire you, and don't be hesitant to seek guidance and assistance when needed. You are not alone on this journey; together, we can overcome any obstacle and attain our objectives.

www.ingramcontent.com/pod-product-compliance
Lightning Source LLC
Chambersburg PA
CBHW051838250726
48659CB00005B/1914